The Essential Keto Diet Book #2021

Lose Weight with Easy and Tasty Weight Loss Recipes incl. 4 Weeks Weight Loss Challenge

David A. Miller

ISBN- 9798563094451

Table of Contents

INTRODUCTION

Are you looking for an effective way to shed those extra pounds and live a healthier lifestyle? The Keto diet could be just what you need. Unlike low calorie and low-fat eating plans, the Keto diet is a long-term solution to losing weight and keeping it off without feeling hungry or unsatisfied.

When you choose a keto lifestyle, you will be able to eat delicious and filling protein packed dishes that help you burn fat more quickly.

A ketogenic diet uses the principle of depleting your body of carbohydrates. These carbs are our primary sources of energy, omitting these from your diet will force your body to burn any fat you have for fuel, this utilises weight loss instantly.

Historically fasting was used to treat various health concerns. Ancient Greek doctors advised restricting your food intake to help treat epilepsy and many other health related diseases. The practice of fasting was kept in record by Hippocrates, and physicians the world over used this practice for many thousands of years.

While many of us will start using a ketogenic diet for weight loss or to make improvements to our health, this eating plan began as a pioneering treatment in epilepsy. It began around 1911 in France, the study showed that if patients adopted a low-calorie diet and combined it with fasting periods, they would experience fewer seizures which helped their overall health conditions.

During that same time period an American Osteopath, Hugh Conklin, also recommended fasting for his patients suffering epilepsy. His method asked for a patient to fast for a period of eighteen to twenty-five days. His conclusions were recorded, and he noted a fifty percent successful outcome for adults and possibly ninety percent in children.

To the world the results were splendid, but a glaring problem was obvious. Whilst fasting controlled seizures, returning to regular eating brought them back.

As many other doctors around the world began having the same results, some decided to experiment and modify the fasts. Focusing to eliminate starches and sugars, instead of restricting calories equally. Doctor Wilder, working at the Mayo Clinic in America, concluded some of his epileptic patients were having fewer seizures if they lowered their blood sugar by eating a high in fat, low in carbohydrates diet. This subsequently created our Keto diet, using the foods to imitate the state of metabolism fasting produces.

After this diet started becoming popular in the treatment of epilepsy, many doctors noticed increased benefits for children. They were observed to be less irritable and more alert which helped in their discipline. Sleeping patterns were more regular which helped with the next day's energy levels.

Despite the many doctor's hard work and proven successes for treating epileptic patients with the keto diet, this way of eating was pushed to the side as drug companies developed anticonvulsant drugs to treat epilepsy. The diet's popularity declined as dieticians were no longer trained to use it. This would subsequently lead to the diet being used incorrectly, giving poor results and being given an ineffective title. After only decades the revolutionary diet was pushed aside for other strategies to tackle epilepsy.

What Should I Know About The Ketogenic Diet?

The basis for trying the ketogenic diet is quite simple. Keeping your body in a fasted state by limiting your carbohydrates will make your body burn fat for fuel, this will maximise your weight loss. Carbohydrates are turned into glucose and we use it for energy, by consuming more fat in your daily diet you will remove sugars from your bloodstream and make your body go into a process called 'Ketosis.' In short, if you follow the keto diet you will convince your body to metabolically act as though it is starving, even though you are consuming enough calories and healthy nutrition to be comfortable.

Dr. Peterman, a well-regarded Mayo Clinic doctor, designed the "classic keto" diet. Today we follow the ratio of 4:1, fats to carbs and proteins. Ninety percent of your calories will come from eating fat, four percent from eating carbohydrates and the remaining six percent protein intake.

The main goal of the keto diet is to restrict the carbs, so our bodies break down the fat for energy. The fats are broken down by the liver, therefore the liver produces ketones. It is then these ketones are used for energy because of the absence of any glucose.

Whilst many keto diets are out there, for you to achieve this state called 'ketosis' you must radically reduce your carbohydrate intake. Our book contains all the recipes you need to help you lose the weight you want and adopt a healthier eating plan. You may also find your appetite becomes suppressed. It is not yet known why this happens but eating less if you are not very active will be beneficial in the long term. You may want to start exercising again as you feel better and slimmer. You may feel your energy levels rise and it could kick start an exercise routine for you. Physical exercise is such an important part of a healthy life, not only for weight loss but for mental health also.

As with any diet plan, always consult your doctor before beginning. Working people with heart disease or at risk of it, are advised against the keto diet. Those with diabetes type two should consult a doctor first. The absence of certain foods and the carbohydrate restriction may be a long-term challenge for some. If you find you are moving from the keto plan to your regular way of eating and back again you will find it much harder to lose the weight you intend to.

Our keto diet plan will be good for you if you are trying to lose excess weight. You will also find the added benefits of being less hungry and having much more energy. This is because you are cutting out the many sugar highs and lows that happen when you are eating very high carbohydrate foods. You will find yourself more alert and able to focus better. Your sleeping pattern will be better, and your clothes will fit again.

How Does The Keto Diet Work?

Unlike many diets now the keto does not have any membership fees or upfront costs. Just commitment and a change to your shopping basket. There are companies out there who will tailor a shopping list and menu for you for a cost. If that is the motivation you need to begin and keep going, then that is a win for yourself. Committing to looking after yourself better takes dedication.

We all know how going on a diet feels like a good idea, you see results and you are looking better. But then you get bored and naughty foods begin slipping back into your shopping basket. Your old habits come back, and the weight goes back on. If you joined a slimming club, you may not want to travel any more or your life changes and you cannot get there every week. If you eat in restaurants a lot you do not always know the ingredients in your dish, or the choices may be poor. Lots of potatoes and rice, pasta dishes with lots of calorie laden sauces.

Processed foods are not part of the keto plan, you will need to buy whole foods, meats and dairy. It may seem to be more expensive at first, but you will soon notice a difference when your kitchen cupboards are full of good nutritious foods that are helping you not only look but feel much better.

You may find yourself buying in bulk and freezing items. If you organise yourself, you will be able to eat nutritious keto friendly foods every day. Make your weekly shopping list according to our recipes, take the time to nourish your body.

Buy fresh in season produce, frozen vegetables will work and are nutritious also. You will find this a good way to keep your costs down. Find a way to bulk buy seeds and nuts. Buy your meat in bulk, portion it accordingly and freeze. Buy the best produce you can afford, especially meat. There are some wonderful butchers and farmers markets around, take the time to find them.

When following the keto plan, you will see it requires you to consume higher amounts of fats, you may wish to substitute some animal fats [because of their high levels they can increase cholesterol] with plant derived fats. Olive oil, avocado oil, sesame oil, are all good and healthy fats for dressings and cooking.

You can incorporate foods with fat rich content, nuts, seeds and avocados are wonderful options. Their benefits include fiber and unsaturated fats. Unfortunately, many fruits are not included or restricted on the keto diet, but no starch, leafy green vegetables will become the core of your eating plan.

Lean protein is the main source of your food, poultry, fish and lean red meat.

Foods you CAN consume on the Keto plan:

VEGETABLES

Non-starchy vegetables are high in nutrients, low in carbs and calories.

- leafy greens, asparagus, cauliflower, cabbage, broccoli, cucumber, green beans, kale, aubergine // eggplant, peppers, spinach, tomatoes, courgettes // zucchini and mushrooms

CHEESE

- high in fats and low in carbs, perfect for the keto plan

DAIRY

- butter, cream, Greek yoghurt, cottage cheese

OLIVE OIL AND COCONUT OIL

MEAT AND POULTRY

Staple foods on the keto plan contain no carbs and are high in protein.

- chicken, pork, turkey, grass fed beef, lamb and game

SEEDS AND NUTS

High fat, low carb snacks

The carbohydrate count per one ounce//28 grams

almonds: 6 grams carbs

Brazil nuts: 3 grams carbs

cashews: 9 grams carbs

macadamia nuts: 4 grams carbs

pecans: 4 grams carbs

pistachios: 8 grams carbs

walnuts: 4 grams carbs

chia seeds: 12 grams carbs

flaxseeds: 8 grams carbs

pumpkin seeds: 5 grams carbs

sesame seeds: 7 grams carbs

FISH AND SHELLFISH

Rich in B vitamins, selenium and potassium

Some shellfish are higher carbs

clams: 4 grams

mussels: 4 grams

octopus: 4 grams

oysters: 3 grams

squid: 3 grams

FRUITS

Most fruits are too high in carbohydrates, berries are the exception.

Strawberries - 4 grams carbs per 50 grams weight

Blackberries - 5 grams carbs per 50 grams weight

Raspberries - 6 grams carbs per 50 grams weight

Blueberries - 6 grams carbs per 50 grams weight

Avocado - 4 grams carbs per 50 grams weight

EGGS

Healthy, nutritious and versatile. High in protein and low in carbs

OLIVES

Rich in antioxidants, delicious and healthy fats

DARK CHOCOLATE AND COCOA POWDER

Dark chocolate is high in antioxidants. Choose over 70% cocoa solids.

COFFEE AND TEA

Drink without any sugar or sweeteners

Green tea

Herbal teas

Foods to avoid and/or limit on the Keto plan:

ALL PROCESSED FOODS

Crackers, crisps // potato chips, corn chips

Ready meals, processed meals

GRAINS

To include:

Bread of any sort

Pasta

Rice

Quinoa

SWEET TREATS

To include:

Cake

Cookies // biscuits

Sweets // candy

STARCHY FOODS

Potatoes

Rice

Couscous

HIGH CARBOHYDRATE FRUITS

To include:

Melons

Tropical fruits

Grapes

Bananas

ARTIFICIAL SWEETENERS

To include:

Splenda

Equal

Aspartame

Saccharin

MARGARINE AND SPREADS

JUICE AND CARBONATED DRINKS

To include:

All carbonated drinks

Fruit juice

Diluting squash drinks

ALCOHOL

As with any new eating plan you decide to try there are always controversies and bad press. For most people the ketogenic diet is a healthy way of eating, weight loss and weight management.

ALWAYS CONSULT YOUR DOCTOR OR DIETICIAN BEFORE STARTING ANY DIET PLAN

Changing Your Habits

So, you have decided you want to lose weight and feel healthier.

Now let us show you how to change your shopping habits and cook the meal you need to keep you on the right path to your weight management goals.

The benefits to you are often similar to the other low carbohydrate diets, but keto will help you burn the fat away and insulin levels will decrease. Helping you stay focused and feeling energetic. Body fat will melt away without you having any hunger pangs.

APPETITE CONTROL

Turning to the keto diet will give you much better control on your appetite.

I'm sure you have tried other diets and always felt hungry, but not with keto and the studies prove it.

With the keto diet you will find the urge to eat less, especially if you wait until the hunger pangs set in before you prepare and eat your food.

It also means you can use intermittent fasting, thus helping speed up your weight loss and reverse any signs of type 2 diabetes.

You may find you begin to save money by not buying lots of snacks and alcohol. Eating twice a day may become your normal.

Sugar addiction is a huge problem in our society, keto will stop those cravings, food will become your friend not your addiction.

GETTING YOUR BODY INTO KETOSIS

Restrict your carbohydrates to 20 grams [digestible] per day. Fiber, however, does not need to be restricted.

No counting of calories needed.

Eat enough recommended fats to make you feel satisfied.

The keto diet is a high-fat plan because those fats are supplying the energy to your body instead of carbohydrates. Once you are feeding your body with those fats you should be into ketosis. You will not feel hungry simply energetic.

Combine your protein packed foods with low carbohydrate vegetables and enough fats to feel you are satisfied.

Protein, you will find, is very filling. You should not be overeating any protein, such as meat and fish.

Avoid snacking. It has probably become a habit, especially if you are somewhere that food is available, and you used to just help yourself. If you do need to snack, eat low starch vegetables in moderation.

If you want to try fasting to accelerate your weight loss you can skip breakfast or dinner and use the time of sleep to add to your fasting time. Make sure you are getting at least seven hours of sleep every night. Manage your stress, hormones produced by stress may increase your blood sugar level, making you want to snack and slowing down your weight loss and ketosis state.

HOW TO TELL YOU ARE IN KETOSIS

You will experience an increase in thirst as your mouth will feel dry. Drink plenty of water. You can drink black coffee and tea and a small amount of bouillon if you need it daily. Your mouth may have a strange metallic taste and your trips to the bathroom to urinate will increase. You may want to test your urine with store bought urine strip tests.

Keto Breath. You may notice your breath has a different smell, it can be fruity or smell similar to nail varnish remover. This is coming from the acetone that our body releases when in ketosis. It is normally temporary.

Reduced appetite. Many will experience a significant hunger reduction whilst following the keto plan.

Possibly an increase in your energy levels. You may feel tired for a few days at first but then your energy will sharply increase.

WHAT CAN I EAT?

How can you start your day? What would you have for breakfast?

If you are a fan of a full cooked breakfast, then this is the plan for you. Eggs, bacon, sausages all a perfect meal to set you up for the day ahead. We also have some delicious meals if you don't want eggs.

Alternatively, if you are not really hungry in the morning and usually do not eat breakfast then just have a drink and use this time to fast.

Now to decide what to have for lunch or dinner. A piece of protein with a side of salad or vegetables. Delicious chicken breast or a fresh piece of tuna. Add the side of your choice a dressing from olive oil and you will be delighted at how easy and simple your food can be.

BUT IT'S SO EXPENSIVE!

It is an untruth that maintaining a keto diet is expensive. You just have to source good quality foods and you will notice a saving on all the nonsense you used to buy.

BREAD

Bread is often a large part of a person's daily intake of food. But don't worry we have plenty of keto bread alternatives.

DINING OUT

You can still visit your favourite restaurants or eat at a friend's house. Just avoid the starchy foods, potatoes, rice, pasta and bread. Choose protein options and ask for your vegetables steamed or sauteed in butter or olive oil. You don't have to miss out!

PACKAGED FOODS

There are many companies selling products aimed at certain diets. Try not to buy and eat these products, they may have hidden carbohydrates in them. Plus, you want to eat as freshly as you can.

LEARN TO ORGANISE YOURSELF

In time you will be so delighted with your weight loss and energy levels, that you will learn to organise your meals, especially if you are working or travelling. Pack up your fresh ingredients or cook the night before, ready to take with you the next day. Plan your shopping list and avoid temptations if you can. Even if you do cheat don't be harsh on yourself, just go back to your plan and stay focused.

HOW CAN I KEEP TRACK OF MY CARBOHYDRATE INTAKE?

By using our recipes and meal plans you can stay below the recommended twenty net grams a day of carbs.

WHAT DO I DO WHEN I REACH MY TARGET WEIGHT?

If you know how much you want to lose and have an end weight in mind, once you reach it you can start to add a few more foods containing carbs. Be mindful that you may gain weight slightly but if you exercise and do not snack you should maintain your goal weight. Learn to love your body and nourish it.

BREAKFASTS

No Bread Sandwich

Serves 1 person

NUTRITION:
Ketogenic low carb
Per serving
Net carbs: 2 % (2 g)
Fiber: 0 g
Fat: 76 % (30 g)
Protein: 23 % (20 g)
kcal: 354

INGREDIENTS:

- 2 tablespoons of butter
- 4 eggs
- Salt, pepper
- 28 grams // 1 oz smoked sliced ham

- 56 grams // 2 oz cheddar, provolone or edam cheese, cut into thick slices
- Tabasco, Worcestershire sauce or mustard to taste

INSTRUCTIONS:

1. Add your two tbsp of butter to your frying pan then put it onto a medium heat. Crack the eggs into the pan and cook on both sides. Add S & P to taste.

2. Using your fried egg for the base of each "sandwich". Layer the meat of your choice onto each stack, then add your cheese choice. Finally, another egg on top. Leave in a warm pan, on a low heat, for the cheese to start melting.

3. Sprinkle with Tabasco, mustard or Worcestershire sauce [if preferred] serve immediately.

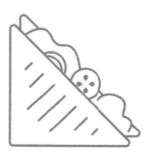

Cheese Crusted Omelette

Serves 1 person

NUTRITION:
Ketogenic low carb
Per serving
Net carbs: 4 % (8 g)
Fiber: 2 g
Fat: 75 % (66 g)
Protein: 21 % (41 g)
kcal: 789

INGREDIENTS:

Omelette

- 2 eggs
- 2 tbsp double/heavy cream
- Salt and pepper

- 1 tablespoon butter or if preferred coconut oil
- 50 grams // ⅓ cup mature grated or sliced cheese

Filling

- 2 sliced mushrooms
- 2 sliced cherry tomatoes
- One tablespoon of baby spinach

- 2 tablespoons of cream cheese
- 25 grams // ⅛ cup turkey slices
- 1 teaspoon dried oregano

INSTRUCTIONS:

1. In a bowl whisk together the cream and eggs. Heat your butter in a frying pan on medium heat. Layer the cheese over the bottom of the frying pan and fry until bubbly.

2. Carefully pour your egg mixture into the pan and turn down the heat. Cook a few minutes, do not stir.

3. Place your mushrooms, spinach, tomatoes, turkey, oregano and cream cheese onto one half of the pan and cook for a while longer.

4. Once the omelette starts to set, turn the other empty half onto the topping side, forming a half moon shape. Cook to your liking and enjoy!

Bacon and Eggs

Serves 4 people

NUTRITION:
Ketogenic low carb
Per serving
Net carbs: 2 % (1 g)
Fiber: 0 g
Fat: 75 % (22 g)
Protein: 23 % (15 g)
kcal: 272

INGREDIENTS:

- 8 eggs
- 140 grams // 5 oz of sliced bacon
- cherry tomatoes
- fresh parsley

INSTRUCTIONS:

1. Place your sliced bacon into your frying pan already warmed to medium heat. Fry to nice and crispy. Take the bacon out of the pan and place aside, leaving the fat in the pan.
2. Crack your eggs into the hot pan and fry eggs however you like them to be. Once your eggs are cooking add the cherry tomatoes and fry all together.
3. Sprinkle with salt and pepper to your liking.

Breakfast Pancakes, Berries and Cream

Serves four people

NUTRITION:
Ketogenic low carb
Per serving
Net carbs: 4 % (4 g)
Fiber: 3 g
Fat: 83 % (39 g)
Protein: 12 % (13 g)
kcal: 424

INGREDIENTS:

Pancakes

- 4 eggs
- 200 grams // ¾ cup of cottage cheese
- 1 tbsp of ground psyllium husk powder
- 50 grams // ¼ cup coconut oil or butter

Toppings

- 50 grams // ¼ cup of berries of your choice
- 230 mls // one cup double/heavy cream

INSTRUCTIONS:

1. Crack the eggs into a large bowl, add your cottage cheese, psyllium husk and mix well together. Let the mixture rest for five to ten minutes or until it thickens up.
2. In a frying pan heat up the coconut oil or butter. Pour dollops of pancake mix into the pan and cook on a medium heat, turning gently until nice and brown on either side.
3. In a separate bowl whisk up the cream to your liking.
4. Serve up your pancakes with cream and the berries you have chosen.

Coconut Pancakes

Serves 4 people

NUTRITION:
Ketogenic low carb
Per serving
Net carbs: 4 % (3 g)
Fiber: 6 g
Fat: 79 % (24 g)
Protein: 17 % (11 g)
kcal: 279

INGREDIENTS:

- 6 eggs
- A pinch of salt
- 2 tbsp coconut oil melted
- 177 mls // ¾ cup coconut milk
- 50 grams // ½ cup coconut flour
- 1 teaspoon baking powder
- Coconut oil or butter, for frying

INSTRUCTIONS:

1. Separate the egg whites and yolks.
2. Whip egg whites with a pinch of salt using your hand mixer. Whip until stiff peaks are formed, set aside.
3. In another bowl, whisk all together the yolks, coconut milk and oil.
4. Add your baking powder to the coconut flour. Then add this to the main bowl and mix gently until a nice smooth batter forms.
5. Gently fold your egg whites mixture into your batter. Let this rest for five minutes.
6. Heat the oil or butter in your frying pan, pour small rounds of your mixture in and cook on each side until nice and brown.
7. Serve immediately.

Banana Waffles

Serves 8 people

NUTRITION:
Liberal low carb
one waffle
Net carbs: 11 % (4 g)
Fiber: 2 g
Fat: 74 % (12 g)
Protein: 14 % (5 g)
kcal: 149

INGREDIENTS:

- One ripened banana
- 4 eggs
- 75 grams // ¾ cup of almond flour
- 175 mls // ¾ cup of coconut milk
- 1 tbsp ground psyllium husk powder
- 1 pinch of salt
- 1 tsp baking powder
- ½ tsp vanilla extract
- 1 tsp of ground cinnamon
- A scoop of coconut oil or butter

INSTRUCTIONS:

1. In a large bowl mix the almond flour, coconut milk, husk powder, salt, baking powder, vanilla extract and cinnamon. Let it sit for half an hour.
2. Set your waffle maker to medium, grease with the coconut oil or butter and once heated pour the batter into the waffle moulds.
3. Cook to your desired colour!
4. Serve with delicious whipped cream and your choice of berries! Happy eating.

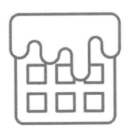

Cauliflower Hash Brown

Serves 4 people

NUTRITION:
Moderate low carb
Per serving
Net carbs: 7 % (5 g)
Fiber: 3 g
Fat: 84 % (26 g)
Protein: 10 % (7 g)
kcal: 282

INGREDIENTS:

- 1 medium cauliflower
- 3 eggs whisked
- ½ yellow onion finely grated
- Black pepper and salt
- 100 grams // ½ cup butter

INSTRUCTIONS:

1. Rinse your cauliflower thoroughly and grate finely either by hand or in an electric food processor.
2. Place your grated cauliflower into a large mixing bowl, add your whisked eggs and the salt and pepper. Mix thoroughly and let it rest for ten minutes.
3. Melt your butter in a large frying pan on a medium heat.
4. Place your first four scoops of pancake mixture into the pan, flatten them down carefully until they are three to four inches diameter.
5. Fry gently for about five minutes each side, adjusting your heat accordingly so they do not burn. Don't be tempted to flip them too early as they will fall apart.
6. Keep your cooked pancakes warm in the oven while you finish your mixture.
7. Serve with homemade mayonnaise or sour cream.

Coconut Porridge

Serves 1 person

NUTRITION:

Ketogenic low carb

Per serving

Net carbs: 3 % (4 g)

Fiber: 5 g

Fat: 90 % (48 g)

Protein: 7 % (9 g)

kcal: 481

INGREDIENTS:

- 1 egg, whisked
- 1 tablespoon coconut flour
- 1 pinch of ground psyllium husk powder
- 1 pinch of salt
- 25 grams // ⅛ cup butter/coconut oil
- 4 tablespoons of coconut cream

INSTRUCTIONS:

1. In your small mixing bowl add the whisked egg, the coconut flour, salt and psyllium husk powder.
2. Place your pan over a medium to low heat, add the coconut cream and butter and melt slowly.
3. Whisk in your egg mixture stirring until you have a thick, creamy texture.
4. Serve with cream and berries or nuts of your choice.

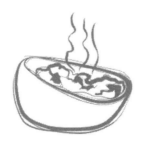

Cheese and Mushroom Fritatta

Serves 4 people

NUTRITION:
Ketogenic low carb
Per serving
Net carbs: 2 % (6 g)
Fiber: 3 g
Fat: 86 % (105 g)
Protein: 12 % (33 g) kcal: 1102

INGREDIENTS:

Frittata

- 440 grams // 1 lb mushrooms
- 110 grams // 4 oz butter
- 6 scallions
- 1 tablespoon fresh parsley
- 1 teaspoon salt
- ½ teaspoon black pepper
- 10 eggs
- 225 grams // 8 oz grated cheese
- 225 mls // 1 cup homemade mayonnaise
- 110 grams // 4 oz leafy greens

Vinaigrette

- 4 tablespoons olive oil
- 1 tablespoon white wine vinegar
- ½ teaspoon salt
- ¼ teaspoon black pepper

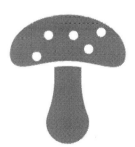

INSTRUCTIONS:

1. Turn your oven on to heat at 175C // 350F.
2. Make your vinaigrette by whisking all the ingredients together in a small jug.
3. Slice up the mushrooms and finely dice the scallions.
4. Place three quarters of the butter to melt in your frying pan on a medium heat.
5. Saute mushroom in your pan until nice and golden in colour.
6. Add the diced scallions into the mushrooms and sprinkle with salt & pepper according to your taste. Add the parsley.
7. Whisk up your eggs, cheese and mayonnaise in a small bowl.
8. Grease a baking dish with the remaining butter.
9. Add your cooked ingredients to the egg mixture and pour into the baking dish.
10. Cook for approximately thirty minutes, the frittata will be a lovely golden colour.
11. Serve with the leafy greens of your choice and vinaigrette.

Scrambled Eggs Mexican Style

Serves 4 people

NUTRITION:
Ketogenic low carb
Per serving
Net carbs: 4 % (2 g)
Fiber: 1 g
Fat: 72 % (18 g)
Protein: 24 % (14 g)
kcal: 229

INGREDIENTS:

- 30 grams // 1 oz butter
- 1 finely chopped scallion
- 2 finely diced pickled jalapeños
- 1 diced tomato
- 6 eggs
- 75 grams // 3 oz grated cheese
- Salt & pepper

INSTRUCTIONS:

1. Melt butter in your frying pan, on medium to high heat.
2. Add the chopped scallions, your diced jalapeños and your diced tomatoes, fry for three to four minutes.
3. Whisk the eggs, pour them into your pan. Cook for two minutes stirring continuously.
4. Add the cheese and salt & pepper to your taste.

Scrambled Eggs and Halloumi Cheese

Serves 2 people

NUTRITION:
Ketogenic low carb
Per serving
Net carbs: 3 % (4 g)
Fiber: 2 g
Fat: 80 % (59 g)
Protein: 17 % (28 g)
kcal: 660

INGREDIENTS:

- 2 tablespoons olive oil
- 75 grams // 3 oz diced halloumi cheese
- 2 chopped scallions,
- 110 grams // 4 oz diced bacon

- 4 tablespoons chopped parsley
- 4 eggs
- Salt & pepper
- 50 grams // 2 oz pitted olives

INSTRUCTIONS:

1. In a medium size frying pan pour the olive oil in to heat. Fry the diced haloumi, diced bacon and the chopped scallions until brown.
2. In a bowl, whisk the parsley with the eggs, salt & pepper.
3. Add this egg mixture to your frying pan covering the bacon, cheese.
4. Turn down the heat, adding the olives, then stir for a few minutes more.

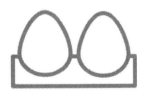

Egg and Chorizo Muffins

Serves 3 people

NUTRITION:
Ketogenic low carb
2 muffins per serving
Net carbs: 2 % (2 g)
Fiber: 0 g
Fat: 69 % (26 g)
Protein: 28 % (24 g)
kcal: 337

INGREDIENTS:

- 1 finely diced scallion
- 75 grams // 3 oz chopped chorizo
- 6 eggs
- 1 tablespoon red pesto
- Salt & pepper
- 75 grams // 3 oz grated cheese

INSTRUCTIONS:

1. Turn on your oven to 175C // 350F.
2. Grease a muffin tin or use paper baking cups.
3. Divide the chorizo and scallions evenly between the cups.
4. In a small bowl whisk the eggs with the pesto and salt & pepper to taste. Add your grated cheese.
5. Pour your mixture into the muffin cups.
6. Cook for fifteen minutes or until set and brown.

Strawberry Smoothie

Serves 2 people

NUTRITION:
Moderate low carb
11 fl. oz or 330 mls
Net carbs: 9 % (10 g)
Fiber: 1 g
Fat: 87 % (42 g)
Protein: 4 % (5 g)
kcal: 418

INGREDIENTS:

♦ 400 grams // 14 fl oz unsweetened coconut milk

♦ 150 grams // 5 oz sliced strawberries

♦ 1 tablespoon lime juice

♦ ½ teaspoon vanilla extract

INSTRUCTIONS:

1. In an electric blender place all your ingredients together.
2. Blend on high until smooth, add lime juice to taste.

Breakfast Oatmeal

Serves 1 person

NUTRITION:
Moderate low carb
Per serving
Net carbs: 5 % (8 g)
Fiber: 8 g
Fat: 88 % (61 g)
Protein: 7 % (10 g) kcal: 615

INGREDIENTS:

- 225 mls // 1 cup canned, unsweetened coconut or almond milk
- 1 tbsp flaxseed, whole
- 1 tbsp chia seeds
- 1 tbsp sunflower seeds
- 1 pinch of salt

INSTRUCTIONS:

1. In a small pan add your ingredients, bringing to a rolling boil.
2. Turn down the heat to let simmer as the mixture thickens.
3. Top with berries or more milk as you need.

Ginger Smoothie

Serves 2 people

NUTRITION:
Liberal low carb
Per serving
Net carbs: 12 % (3 g)
Fiber: 1 g
Fat: 81 % (8 g)
Protein: 6 % (1 g)
kcal: 82

INGREDIENTS:

- 75 mls // 1/3 cup of coconut milk/ coconut cream
- 150 mls // 2/4 cup of water
- 2 tablespoons lime juice
- 30 grams // 1 oz frozen spinach
- 2 teaspoons freshly grated ginger

INSTRUCTIONS:

1. Mix everything together in an electric blender.
2. Use lime juice to taste.

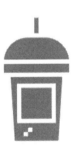

Tofu Vegan Scramble

Serves 2 people

NUTRITION:
Moderate low carb
Per serving
Net carbs: 3 % (2 g)
Fiber: 5 g
Fat: 51 % (17 g)
Protein: 46 % (35 g)
kcal: 281

INGREDIENTS:

- 375 grams // 13 oz firm tofu
- ¼ teaspoon turmeric
- 1 tablespoon nutritional yeast
- 175 mls // ¾ cup almond milk, unsweetened
- Salt & pepper
- 1 tablespoon finely chopped chives

INSTRUCTIONS:

1. Cut the tofu into medium sized pieces.
2. Heat a frying pan and add the tofu on a medium heat.
3. Add the turmeric and yeast, stirring well. Cook for five minutes.
4. Pour over your almond milk, simmering for another ten minutes. Occasionally stir, season with salt and pepper and your chives.

English Muffins

Serves 3 people

NUTRITION:
Ketogenic low carb
Per serving
Net carbs: 2 % (1 g)
Fiber: 2 g
Fat: 86 % (15 g)
Protein: 12 % (5 g)
kcal: 156

INGREDIENTS:

- 2 eggs
- 2 tablespoons coconut flour
- ½ teaspoon baking powder
- 1 pinch of salt
- 3 tablespoons of butter/ coconut oil

INSTRUCTIONS:

1. In a bowl mix the coconut flour, salt and baking powder.
2. Add the eggs and whisk all together. Let it rest for a minute.
3. Heat your frying pan and add the butter or oil on a medium heat.
4. Dollop your batter into the pan and cook. Turning as they brown.
5. Serve with your favourite toppings.

Granola

Serves 5 people

NUTRITION:

Moderate low carb

Calculations based on 1 serving of granola served with 🄰 cup of full-fat Greek yogurt.

Net carbs: 8 % (7 g)

Fiber: 5 g

Fat: 73 % (29 g)

Protein: 18 % (16 g)

kcal: 357

INGREDIENTS:

- 50 grams // 2 oz pecans, hazelnuts or chopped almonds
- 25 grams // 1 oz finely shredded coconut
- 35 grams // ¼ cup sunflower seeds
- 1 tablespoon pumpkin seeds
- 1 tablespoon sesame seeds
- 3 tablespoons flaxseed
- ¼ tablespoon turmeric
- ¼ tablespoon ground cinnamon
- ½ teaspoon vanilla extract
- 2 tablespoons almond flour
- 60 mls // ¼ cup water
- 1 tablespoon coconut oil

INSTRUCTIONS:

1. Turn on your oven and set to 300F // 150C.
2. In an electric food processor add the nuts and blend until they are just chopped.
3. In a bowl add the nuts and all the rest of the ingredients.
4. Line your baking tray with parchment paper and spread the nutty mixture out onto it evenly.
5. Put into your oven and cook for twenty minutes exactly.
6. Do not burn.
7. Take out of the oven and stir around, put back into oven for another twenty minutes.
8. Once the granola is feeling dry turn off your oven but leave the tray inside the oven to finish off.
9. Take out and serve with your choice of accompaniment. Greek yogurt or cream and berries would be a delicious start to your day.

Keto Bread

Serves 6 people

NUTRITION:
Ketogenic low carb
1 bun is 1 serving
Net carbs: 4 % (2 g)
Fiber: 7 g
Fat: 78 % (12 g)
Protein: 17 % (6 g)
kcal: 164

INGREDIENTS:

- 5 tablespoons ground psyllium husk powder
- 150 grams // 1 ¼ cup almond flour
- 2 teaspoons baking powder
- 1 teaspoon sea salt
- 225 mls // 1 cup water
- 2 teaspoons cider vinegar
- 3 egg whites
- 2 tablespoons sesame seeds

INSTRUCTIONS:

1. Heat the oven at 350F // 175C.
2. In your large bowl mix up the dry ingredients.
3. Bring the measured water to the boil.
4. Whisk the egg whites with the vinegar and add this to your dry ingredients, mixing it all well.
5. Be careful not to mix too much, it should be like play dough.
6. Grease a baking tray.
7. Wet your hands with some olive oil.
8. Shape your dough into six rolls and put onto your baking tray, sprinkle sesame seeds over the top.
9. Place the tray onto the lowest rack of your oven and cook for an hour.
10. Serve fresh with your choice of toppings.

Cloud Bread

Serves 4 people

NUTRITION:
Moderate low carb
Per serving
Net carbs: 5 % (2 g)
Fiber: 1 g
Fat: 79 % (14 g)
Protein: 15 % (6 g)
kcal: 162

INGREDIENTS:

- 3 eggs
- 125 grams // 4 ½ oz of cream cheese
- A pinch of salt
- ½ tablespoon ground psyllium husk powder
- ½ teaspoon baking powder
- ¼ teaspoon cream of tartar

INSTRUCTIONS:

1. Separate your egg whites from your egg yolks.
2. Whisk the egg whites with salt until they are very stiff. Turn your bowl over to check, the whites should not move.
3. In your other bowl add the cream cheese to the egg yolks and mix together. You can add your baking powder and psyllium husk powder at this point if you wish to give your cloud bread a more dough like consistency.
4. With great care fold your egg whites in with your egg yolk mixture, keeping them full of air.
5. Line a baking tray with greaseproof paper.
6. Evenly drop spoonfuls of your mixture onto the tray, making sure you have room to make them circles with a spoon.
7. Heat your oven to 150C // 300F.
8. Put into the oven and cook for approximately 25 minutes, they will be a nice golden brown.

BLT Sandwich Made With Cloud Bread

Serves 2 people

NUTRITION:
Ketogenic low carb
Per serving
Net carbs: 4 % (7 g)
Fiber: 3 g
Fat: 83 % (65 g)
Protein: 13 % (22 g)
kcal: 705

INGREDIENTS:

- 2 tablespoons homemade mayonnaise
- 150 grams // 5 oz lean bacon
- 50 grams // 2 oz lettuce
- 1 thinly sliced beefsteak tomato

INSTRUCTIONS:

1. Fry your bacon in a frying pan until nice and crispy.
2. Take two pieces of cloud bread and spread your mayonnaise onto one piece.
3. Layer with tomato and lettuce then top with the other piece of cloud bread.

Chai Tea

Serves 2 people

NUTRITION:
Ketogenic low carb
Per serving
Net carbs: 3 % (1 g)
Fiber: 0 g
Fat: 94 % (14 g)
Protein: 3 % (1 g)
kcal: 133

INGREDIENTS:

- 1 tablespoon chai tea
- 475 mls // 2 cups water
- 75 mls // 1/3 cup double cream

INSTRUCTIONS:

1. Brew your tea according to package instructions.
2. Warm the cream, add to your tea before enjoying!

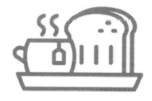

LUNCHES

Antipasto Salad

Serves 2 people

NUTRITION:
Moderate low carb
Per serving
Net carbs: 6 % (13 g)
Fiber: 9 g
Fat: 74 % (65 g)
Protein: 19 % (38 g)
kcal: 823

INGREDIENTS:

- 275 grams // 10oz Romaine lettuce finely chopped
- 2 tablespoons chopped parsley
- 150 grams // 5 oz sliced mozzarella cheese
- 75 grams // 3 oz Parma ham
- 75 grams // 3 oz thinly sliced salami
- 150 grams // 5 oz can of artichoke in water, drain and quarter
- 75 grams // 3 oz jar of drained roast red peppers
- 30 grams // 1 oz chopped sun-blush tomatoes
- 30 grams // 1 oz sliced olives
- Bunch of fresh basil
- 1 de-seeded and diced red chili pepper
- ½ tablespoon sea salt
- 4 tablespoons olive oil

INSTRUCTIONS:

1. Wash the lettuce and chop into small pieces.
2. Arrange lettuce onto your large platter.
3. Sprinkle the parsley and begin to layer up the antipasto ingredients.
4. Combine chilli pepper, basil and salt together.
5. Sprinkle this over your salad and finally drizzle the olive oil.

Smoked Salmon With Avocado

Serves 2 people

NUTRITION:
Ketogenic low carb
Per serving
Net carbs: 2 % (4 g)
Fiber: 13 g
Fat: 86 % (75 g)
Protein: 12 % (23 g)
kcal: 811

INGREDIENTS:

- 200 grams // 8 oz of smoked salmon
- 2 avocados
- 125 mls // ½ cup of homemade mayonnaise
- Salt & pepper

INSTRUCTIONS:

1. Cut the avocado in two and remove the stone.
2. Scoop the fruit out with a spoon onto your plate.
3. Arrange the smoked salmon and mayonnaise on the plate, season to taste with salt & pepper.

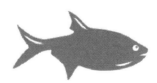

Feta Cheese With Chicken Salad

Serves 2 people

NUTRITION:
Ketogenic low carb
Per serving
Net carbs: 3 % (10 g)
Fiber: 4 g
Fat: 76 % (103 g)
Protein: 21 % (63 g)
kcal: 1212

INGREDIENTS:

- 450 grams // 1 lb Roast chicken
- 200 grams // 7 oz feta cheese
- 2 tomatoes
- 475 mls // 2 cups leafy greens
- 10 black pitted olives
- 75 mls // ⅓ cup olive oil
- Salt & pepper

INSTRUCTIONS:

1. Slice your tomatoes, arrange with the chicken, cheese and lettuce and olives onto your plate.
2. Season to taste, drizzle with your olive oil.

Pesto Chicken and Zoodle Salad

Serves 4 people

NUTRITION:
Ketogenic low carb
Per serving
Net carbs: 3 % (5 g)
Fiber: 2 g
Fat: 76 % (51 g)
Protein: 21 % (32 g)
kcal: 616

INGREDIENTS:

- 600 grams // 1 1/3 lbs boneless and skinless chicken thighs
- 75 mls // 1/3 cup homemade green pesto
- 150 grams // 5 oz roughly chopped cherry tomatoes
- 110 grams // 4 oz feta cheese
- 350 grams // 12 oz courgette/zucchini
- 3 tablespoons olive oil

INSTRUCTIONS:

1. In a medium sized pot place chicken thighs. Add water until covered and bring to a rolling boil.
2. Reduce your heat, simmering for fifteen minutes or cooked thoroughly.
3. Drain the chicken thighs then shred the meat. Set aside.
4. Use a spiralizer to make the zucchini/courgette zoodles.
5. Place your zoodles into a large bowl and pour over your pesto. Mix together to thoroughly coat using tongs.
6. Add your chicken and tomatoes and feta. Drizzle with your oil and combine.

Avocado and Seafood Salad

Serves 6 people

NUTRITION:
Ketogenic low carb
Per serving
Net carbs: 3 % (3 g)
Fiber: 2 g
Fat: 71 % (33 g)
Protein: 26 % (27 g)
kcal: 427

INGREDIENTS:

Salad dressing

- 2 tablespoons of lime juice
- 125 mls // ½ cup homemade mayonnaise
- 75 mls // ⅓ cup sour cream
- 1 minced garlic clove
- 1 teaspoon salt
- 60 mls // ¼ cup finely diced red onions
- ¼ teaspoon white pepper

Seafood salad

- 450 grams // 1 lb cooked shrimp
- 450 grams // 1 lb cooked salmon fillets
- 75 grams // 2 ½ oz diced tomatoes
- 40 grams // 1 ½ oz chopped and deseeded cucumber
- 1 avocado
- 2 tablespoons fresh basil, torn into pieces

INSTRUCTIONS:

1. Make your dressing first. In a bowl combine your mayonnaise, garlic, lime juice, diced red onions, sour cream and salt. Put to one side.
2. Chop up your salmon and shrimp. Arrange on your plate along with the tomato, cucumber and avocado.
3. Pour the dressing over your fish and salad and gently mix to coat.
4. Chill for half an hour before serving.

Roast Beef With Cheddar Cheese Salad

Serves 2 people

NUTRITION:

Ketogenic low carb

Per serving

Net carbs: 2 % (6 g)

Fiber: 8 g

Fat: 83 % (98 g)

Protein: 14 % (38 g)

kcal: 1073

INGREDIENTS:

- 200 grams // 8 oz sliced cold roast beef
- 150 grams // 5 oz cheddar cheese
- 1 avocado
- 6 radishes
- 1 scallion
- 125 mls // ½ cup homemade mayonnaise
- 1 tablespoon Dijon mustard
- 50 grams // 2 oz lettuce
- 2 tablespoons olive oil
- Salt & pepper

INSTRUCTIONS:

1. Arrange the meat and cheese, the avocado and radishes onto a plate. Sprinkle on your sliced scallions.
2. Add mayonnaise and mustard.
3. Serve with olive oil and lettuce of your choice.

Cauliflower Cheese

Serves 6 people

NUTRITION:
Moderate low carb
Per serving
Net carbs: 9 % (11 g)
Fiber: 5 g
Fat: 78 % (44 g)
Protein: 13 % (17 g)
kcal: 511

INGREDIENTS:

- 450 grams // 1lb broccoli florets
- 200 grams // 7 oz cream cheese
- 225 mls // 1 cup double cream
- 50 grams // 2 oz butter
- Salt & pepper

- 2 teaspoons garlic powder
- 800 grams // 1 ¾ lbs chopped cauliflower
- 225 grams // 8 oz grated cheese

INSTRUCTIONS:

1. Turn on the oven to 180C // 350F.
2. Steam the broccoli florets in your steamer pan until al dente.
3. In a large bowl puree cream, cream cheese, butter, garlic powder, salt and pepper until smooth. Add the steamed broccoli to this mixture then puree again.
4. Grease your baking dish of choice with butter.
5. Chop up the cauliflower into florets and place in your dish.
6. Pour your creamy broccoli sauce over the top of the cauliflower and sprinkle with grated cheese.
7. Bake in your pre heated oven for forty minutes until golden brown.

Goats Cheese And Spinach Pie

Serves 6 people

NUTRITION:
Ketogenic low carb
Per serving
Net carbs: 3 % (4 g)
Fiber: 3 g
Fat: 82 % (57 g)
Protein: 15 % (23 g)
kcal: 629

INGREDIENTS:

Pie crust

- 150 grams // 1 ¼ cups almond flour
- 3 tablespoons sesame seeds
- 1 tablespoon ground psyllium husk powder
- ½ teaspoon salt
- 40 grams // 1 ½ oz butter
- 1 egg

Egg Batter

- 5 eggs
- 225 mls // 1 cup double cream or use sour cream
- Salt & pepper

Spinach and Goat Cheese Filling

- 200 grams // 7 oz chopped spinach leaves
- 2 tablespoons butter/coconut oil
- 1 garlic clove
- 1 pinch of ground nutmeg
- Salt & pepper
- 100 grams // 1 cup grated cheese
- 175 grams // 6 oz sliced goats cheese

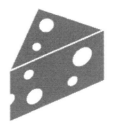

INSTRUCTIONS:

1. Turn your oven on to 175C // 350F.
2. To make the pie crust. In an electric blender mix up your almond flour with the sesame seeds. Add the rest of the ingredients and pulse to get a dough.
3. Roll out the dough and press it into your springform baking pan, use a fork to prick holes for better crust.
4. Blind bake for ten to fifteen minutes.
5. Whisk your eggs with your choice of cream, season with salt & pepper.
6. In a frying pan saute the diced garlic in oil and add spinach. Stir constantly, season.
7. Add this spinach and garlic into the pie crust.
8. Add your cheese into the egg and cream mix and pour this into your pie.
9. Sprinkle with your goats cheese.
10. Bake in the oven for thirty to forty minutes.

Turnip Gratin

Serves 4 people

NUTRITION:
Moderate low carb
Per serving
Net carbs: 8 % (8 g)
Fiber: 2 g
Fat: 81 % (35 g)
Protein: 11 % (11 g)
kcal: 387

INGREDIENTS:

- 1 small onion
- 450 grams // 1lb turnip
- 1 garlic clove
- 75 mls // ⅓ cup fresh chopped chives
- 40 grams // ⅛ cup butter
- 200 mls // ¾ cup double cream
- 125 grams // 1 cup cheese
- ⅓ teaspoon salt
- Pinch of black pepper

INSTRUCTIONS:

1. Turn on your oven to 200C // 400F.
2. Peel your garlic, onion and turnip. Slice them as thinly as you can. Use a mandolin if you have one.
3. Finely chop up the chives.
4. Grease your baking dish of choice with butter.
5. Alternate the slices of cut vegetables, chives and cheese [save a bit for the top].
6. Season with salt & pepper.
7. Pour the double cream onto this and sprinkle the remaining cheese to top.
8. Bake in your hot oven for thirty minutes, it will be bubbling and golden in colour.

Sugar Snap Pea And Roasted Fennel Salad

Serves 4 people

NUTRITION:
Liberal low carb
Per serving
Net carbs: 19 % (8 g)
Fiber: 5 g
Fat: 71 % (12 g)
Protein: 10 % (4 g)
kcal: 165

INGREDIENTS:

- 450 grams // 1lb fresh fennel
- 3 tablespoons olive oil
- Sea salt
- Black pepper
- 1 lemon
- 2 tbsp pumpkin or toasted sunflower seeds
- 150 grams // 5 oz sugar snap peas

INSTRUCTIONS:

1. Heat your oven to 225C // 450F.
2. Cut the fronds and stalks from the fennel bulb and cut into quite small wedges. Place them into your baking dish, drizzling with olive oil and season.
3. Halve the lemon and squeeze the juice out.
4. Peel some lemon rind and put with the fennel.
5. Bake in your oven for twenty to thirty minutes, the fennel will be a golden colour.
6. While this is baking in the oven, toast your pumpkin seeds using your dry pan over a medium heat only for a couple of minutes, do not burn them.
7. Once the fennel is cooked mix it together with your pumpkin seeds and sugar snap peas. Arrange on your plate and enjoy.

Baked Bell Peppers

Serves 4 people

NUTRITION:

Moderate low carb

Per serving

Net carbs: 6 % (6 g)

Fiber: 1 g

Fat: 82 % (37 g)

Protein: 12 % (12 g)

kcal: 412

INGREDIENTS:

- 8 small bell peppers
- 30 grams // 1 oz chopped chorizo
- 1 tablespoon chopped thyme
- 225 grams // 8 oz cream cheese
- ½ tablespoon mild chipotle paste
- 2 tablespoons olive oil
- 110 grams // 4 oz grated cheese

INSTRUCTIONS:

1. Heat your oven to 200C // 325F.
2. Cut your peppers lengthwise then remove the inside core and seeds.
3. Mix together the chorizo and herbs.
4. In another bowl combine cream cheese, olive oil and chipotle paste. Add in your chorizo, herb mix and stir together until smooth.
5. Stuff your peppers with this mixture and put into your greased cooking dish.
6. Sprinkle cheese over the top and bake in your oven for twenty minutes. The cheese will be melted and brown in colour.

Tortilla Pizzas

Serves 4 people

NUTRITION:
Moderate low carb
Per serving
Net carbs: 5 % (5 g)
Fiber: 2 g
Fat: 74 % (33 g)
Protein: 21 % (21 g)
kcal: 410

INGREDIENTS:

Topping

- ♦ 125 mls // ½ cup of tomato sauce
- ♦ 225 grams // 8 oz grated cheese
- ♦ 2 teaspoons dried basil / oregano
- ♦ Salt & pepper

Low-carbohydrate tortillas

- ♦ 2 eggs
- ♦ 2 egg whites
- ♦ 175 grams // 6 oz cream cheese
- ♦ ¼ teaspoon salt
- ♦ 1 teaspoon ground psyllium husk powder
- ♦ 1 tablespoon coconut flour

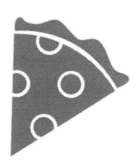

INSTRUCTIONS:

1. Heat your oven to 200C // 400F.
2. Crack your eggs into a bowl and whisk until thick and fluffy. Add your cream cheese and whisk to a smooth consistency.
3. Put your coconut flour, salt and psyllium husk into a bowl and combine.
4. Add your flour mix small amounts in a time to the egg batter and keep whisking. Once finished it will be like breakfast pancake batter.
5. Line 2 baking sheets with baking paper. Spread your batter thinly into tortilla shapes and bake on the top rack quickly for about five minutes. It will be brown round the edges.
6. Turn the oven up - 225C // 450F.
7. Take each tortilla and spread one tbsp of your tomato paste onto each one.
8. Sprinkle with the herbs and cheese.
9. Bake in the very hot oven, watch as the cheese melts.
10. Enjoy!

Broccoli and Kale Salad

Serves 2 people

NUTRITION:
Moderate low carb
Per serving
Net carbs: 6 % (14 g)
Fiber: 19 g
Fat: 86 % (94 g)
Protein: 9 % (22 g)
kcal: 1026

INGREDIENTS:

- 125 mls // ½ cup homemade mayonnaise
- 1 tablespoon grain mustard
- 4 eggs
- 2 avocados
- 2 garlic cloves

- 225 grams // 8 oz chopped broccoli
- 110 grams // 4 oz chopped kale
- 2 sliced scallions
- 2 tablespoons olive oil
- 1 pinch of chilli flakes
- Salt & pepper

INSTRUCTIONS:

1. Mix the mayonnaise and mustard.
2. Boil eggs how you want them. Immediately plunge into cold iced water. Once they have cooled, take the shells off and cut into quarters.
3. Peel and slice the garlic cloves and saute in oil in your frying pan. Do not burn.
4. Remove and crisp them on a piece of paper towel.
5. Add the butter to the oil in the frying pan and saute the chopped kale, broccoli and sliced scallions for 2 minutes, they will be softer.
6. Turn the vegetables onto your plate along with the eggs and avocado. Dollop mustard mayonnaise over the top and sprinkle your crispy garlic slices to give lots of crunch and flavour.

Walnut And Courgette // Zucchini Salad

Serves 4 people

NUTRITION:
Moderate low carb
Per serving
Net carbs: 5 % (7 g)
Fiber: 7 g
Fat: 90 % (58 g)
Protein: 6 % (8 g)
kcal: 584

INGREDIENTS:

Dressing

- 2 tablespoons olive oil
- 175 mls // ¾ cup homemade mayonnaise
- 2 teaspoons lemon juice
- 1 minced garlic clove
- ½ teaspoon salt
- ¼ teaspoon chilli powder

Salad

- 1 Romaine lettuce
- 110 grams // 1 cup rocket/arugula leaves
- 60 mls // ¼ cup finely chopped chives
- 2 courgettes/zucchini
- 1 tablespoon olive oil
- Salt & pepper
- 100 grams // ¾ cup chopped walnuts

INSTRUCTIONS:

1. In a jug whisk the dressing ingredients together.
2. Chop up the lettuce leaves to your liking. Place them along with the chives into your salad bowl.
3. Cut the courgettes/zucchini length wise, scooping out any seeds. Chop into smaller pieces.
4. In your frying pan heat up the oil over a medium heat.
5. Add the chopped courgettes/zucchini and saute until still firm but browned. Season to taste.
6. Place those vegetables into the salad bowl with the leaves, drizzle your dressing over and toss.
7. Quickly roast the walnuts in the hot frying pan and finish off the salad with them.

DINNER RECIPES

Garlic Chicken

Serves 4 people

NUTRITION:
Ketogenic low carb
Per serving
Net carbs: 2 % (3 g)
Fiber: 1 g
Fat: 66 % (39 g)
Protein: 31 % (42 g)
kcal: 542

INGREDIENTS:

- 50 grams // 2 oz butter
- 900 grams // 2 lbs chicken drumsticks or thighs
- Salt & pepper
- 1 lemon
- 2 tablespoons olive oil
- 7 minced garlic cloves
- 30 grams // ½ cup finely chopped parsley

INSTRUCTIONS:

1. Turn on the oven to 225C // 450F.
2. Place your chicken pieces in a large plastic ziplock bag.
3. Add the seasoning, the garlic, olive oil, parsley and lemon juice. Shake vigorously until well coated.
4. Empty into a baking dish and cook in the oven for about forty minutes. Lower the oven temperature and finish cooking until golden brown.

Coconut Curried Chicken

Serves 4 people

NUTRITION:
Ketogenic low carb
Per serving
Net carbs: 4 % (8 g)
Fiber: 5 g
Fat: 79 % (70 g)
Protein: 17 % (33 g)
kcal: 793

INGREDIENTS:

- 2 lemongrass stalks
- 2 tablespoons coconut oil
- 1 tablespoon curry powder
- 650 grams // 1 ½ lbs boneless and skinless chicken thighs
- 1 leek

- 1 piece fresh ginger
- 2 chopped garlic cloves
- 1 sliced red pepper
- ½ finely diced red chilli pepper
- 400 grams // 14 oz coconut milk
- 1 lime, grated zest

INSTRUCTIONS:

1. Take your lemongrass stalk and crush it with the side of your cooking knife.
2. Chop the chicken into pieces.
3. Heat up your coconut oil gently in your wok or frying pan.
4. Grate your ginger and saute with your lemongrass and the curry powder.
5. To the pan, add roughly ½ of your chicken, cook on a medium heat, the chicken will become nice and golden.
6. Set to one side and continue to cook the remaining chicken pieces, leaving the lemongrass in your pan. When finished, place all cooked chicken together.
7. Slice up the leeks and add to the pan with the peppers and chopped garlic. Saute for five minutes. Return the chicken to the pan adding the coconut milk, simmer for five to ten minutes allowing the flavours to fuse together.
8. Remove the lemongrass and finish with grated lime zest.

Thai Flavoured Fish Curry

Serves 4 people

NUTRITION:
Ketogenic low carb
Per serving
Net carbs: 4 % (10 g)
Fiber: 5 g
Fat: 80 % (90 g)
Protein: 16 % (42 g)
kcal: 1014

INGREDIENTS:

- 50 grams // 2 oz coconut oil
- 650 grams // 1 ½ lbs fish (cod or salmon)
- Salt & pepper
- 50 grams // 2 oz butter
- 2 tablespoons red/green Thai curry paste
- 475 mls // 2 cups coconut milk
- 125 mls // ½ cup chopped coriander/cilantro
- 450 grams // 1 lb of cauliflower/broccoli

INSTRUCTIONS:

1. Turn on your oven and set it to 200C // 400F.
2. Grease your baking dish with the coconut oil.
3. Place fish of your choosing into baking dish, pop a small amount of butter onto each piece. Season.
4. In a small bowl mix together the coconut milk, chopped coriander/cilantro and curry paste of your choosing.
5. Pour this mixture over the fish.
6. Put your dish into cook for twenty minutes, test with a knife to make sure it is cooked.
7. Steam your choice of broccoli or cauliflower until al dente, serve with your curried fish.

Oriental Stir Fry With Cabbage

Serves 4 people

NUTRITION:
Ketogenic low carb
Per serving
Net carbs: 4 % (9 g)
Fiber: 4 g
Fat: 83 % (86 g)
Protein: 13 % (31 g)
kcal: 943

INGREDIENTS:

Stir Fry

- 450 grams // 1lb green cabbage
- 110 grams // 4 oz butter
- 1 teaspoon salt
- 1 teaspoon onion powder
- ¼ teaspoon black pepper
- 1 tablespoon white wine vinegar
- 2 minced garlic cloves

- 1 teaspoon chilli flakes
- 50 grams // 2 oz fresh ginger
- 550 grams // 1 ¼ lbs minced/ground beef
- 3 scallions
- 1 tablespoon sesame oil

Wasabi mayonnaise

- 225 mls // 1 cup homemade mayonnaise
- ½ tablespoon wasabi paste

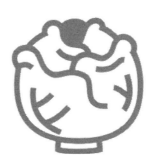

INSTRUCTIONS:

1. Finely slice up the cabbage.

2. Heat half the amount of butter in your wok or frying pan and add the cabbage, saute at a medium heat. This will take a while, do not let it burn.

3. Add the spices with the vinegar to the pan and cook for a few minutes more.

4. Place the spiced cabbage into your bowl.

5. Add the remaining butter to your pan. Saute the diced garlic, grated ginger and chilli flakes.

6. Add your minced beef and cook thoroughly, the juice will evaporate.

7. Turn down the heat on the pan and add the sliced scallions and spiced cabbage to your meat. Stir to mix everything together, season and drizzle sesame oil just before serving.

8. Mix your wasabi mayonnaise ingredients together and serve with your stir fry.

Chinese Style Pork Belly and Brussels Sprouts

Serves 2 people

NUTRITION:
Ketogenic low carb
Per serving
Net carbs: 3 % (7 g)
Fiber: 5 g
Fat: 89 % (97 g)
Protein: 8 % (19 g)
kcal: 993

INGREDIENTS:

- 300 grams // 2/3 lb pork belly
- 1 tablespoon tamari /soy sauce
- ½ tablespoon rice vinegar
- 1 minced garlic clove

- 40 grams // ⅓ cup butter / coconut oil
- 225 grams // ½ lb Brussels sprouts
- ¼ leek

INSTRUCTIONS:

1. Dice up the pork belly to your liking.
2. Rinse the Brussels, trim and quarter.
3. Heat your pan and add the pork pieces, cooking on a medium heat, saute until a golden brown colour.
4. Add the minced garlic, butter or oil and your Brussel sprouts and leeks. Cook until your vegetables are still al dente, but golden brown.
5. In a bowl mix up your soy sauce with the rice vinegar, add this mixture to your pan.
6. Season and serve.

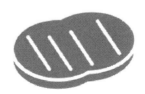

Pork Chops and Blue Cheese Sauce

Serves 4 people

NUTRITION:
Ketogenic low carb
Per serving
Net carbs: 2 % (4 g)
Fiber: 1 g
Fat: 70 % (60 g)
Protein: 28 % (54 g)
kcal: 779

INGREDIENTS:

- 150 grams // 5 oz blue cheese
- 85 grams // ¾ cup double cream
- 4 medium sized pork chops
- Salt & pepper
- 200 grams // 7 oz fine green beans

INSTRUCTIONS:

1. In a small pan crumble the blue cheese, on a medium heat setting. Adjust your heat to allow it to melt gently. Do not allow it to burn.
2. Once this has melted add your cream and simmer for two minutes.
3. Season your pork chops and fry on a medium heat for three minutes each side. Make sure they are thoroughly cooked without drying them out.
4. Cover with some foil and put aside.
5. Add any pan juices to your cheese sauce, stir and heat if needed.
6. Saute or steam your fine green beans as to your liking. Season.

Smoked Ham And Courgette // Zucchini

Serves 4 people

NUTRITION
Moderate low carb
200 g zucchini per serving
Net carbs: 5 % (6 g)
Fiber: 2 g
Fat: 70 % (39 g)
Protein: 25 % (32 g)
kcal: 505

INGREDIENTS:

- 2 courgettes/zucchini
- 1 teaspoon salt
- 1 tablespoon olive oil
- 400 grams // 15 oz smoked ham
- 110 grams // 4 oz cottage cheese
- 2 tablespoons homemade mayonnaise
- 2 tablespoons diced red onions

- ½ tablespoon dried rosemary
- 175 grams // 6 oz grated cheese
- Salt & pepper
- 200 grams // 2 cups lettuce
- 4 tablespoons olive oil
- ½ tablespoon white wine vinegar

INSTRUCTIONS:

1. Heat your oven to 200C // 400F.
2. Cut the courgettes/zucchini into halves lengthwise. Remove seeds and season with salt. Leave for ten minutes.
3. Pat dry and put into your already greased baking dish.
4. Cut up your ham and combine it with the cottage cheese, diced red onion, mayonnaise and rosemary.
5. Add one third of the cheese and season.
6. Divide this mix between the courgette/zucchini halves, top with the rest of your cheese. Bake for half an hour until they look golden brown.
7. Make your vinaigrette for your lettuce salad. Serve together.

Swedish Meatballs

Serves 4 people

NUTRITION:
Moderate low carb
Per serving
Net carbs: 5 % (9 g)
Fiber: 3 g
Fat: 79 % (66 g)
Protein: 16 % (31 g)
kcal: 757

INGREDIENTS:

Meatballs

- ½ onion
- 450 grams // 1 lb minced beef or pork, or both combined
- 110 grams // 4 oz cream cheese
- 1 egg

- 1 teaspoon salt
- 1 pinch of pepper
- 1 pinch of ground allspice
- 3 tablespoons butter

Cream sauce

- 300 mls // 1 ¼ cups double cream
- 50 grams // 2 oz cream cheese

- 450 grams // 15 oz cauliflower
- 4 tablespoons cranberries

INSTRUCTIONS:

1. Finely chop up the onion and place into your mixing bowl.
2. Add the minced meat and other meatball ingredients.
3. With wet hands start rolling the mixture into one inch in size balls.
4. Heat the butter in your frying pan, cook the meatballs on a medium heat until cooked thoroughly.
5. In a separate pan warm the cream cheese with the cream. Add any juice left over from your frying pan, use water to dilute if the sauce is too thick. Season to adjust taste.
6. Steam the cauliflower.
7. Heat up the cranberries, adding honey if needed to sweeten.
8. Serve all together.

The Best Lasagne

Serves 6 people
NUTRITION:
Ketogenic low carb
Per serving
Net carbs: 4 % (8 g)
Fiber: 8 g
Fat: 73 % (60 g)
Protein: 22 % (41 g)
kcal: 756

INGREDIENTS:

Lasagne sheets

- 8 eggs
- 275 grams // 10 oz cream cheese
- 1 teaspoon salt
- 50 grams // ⅓ cup ground psyllium husk powder
- Meat sauce
- 3 tablespoons olive oil
- ½ chopped onion

- 1 minced garlic clove
- 650 grams // 1 ½ lbs minced beef
- 2 tablespoons tomato paste
- ½ tablespoon dried basil
- 1 teaspoon salt
- ¼ teaspoon black pepper
- 125 mls // ½ cup water

Cheese topping

- 350 mls // 1 ½ cups sour cream
- 100 grams // 1 cup grated mozzarella cheese
- 40 grams // ½ cup grated Parmesan cheese
- ½ teaspoon salt
- ¼ teaspoon black pepper
- 30 grams // ½ cup chopped fresh parsley

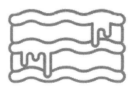

INSTRUCTIONS:

1. Turn on your oven and heat to 150C // 300F. Line your baking sheet with baking paper.

2. Whisk your ingredients together in a bowl until smooth. Whisk the psyllium husk in gradually and place to one side.

3. Pour the mixture onto the middle of the baking paper, put another piece of paper on top and flatten out to form the lasagne sheets. If you feel the pasta sheets are too thick make two batches.

4. Keep the baking paper on and bake in the oven for ten minutes. Put to one side to cool down. Once cool, remove the paper sheet and slice to fit your baking dish.

5. Place the olive oil in your frying pan over a medium heat. Saute the garlic and onion until soft.

6. Add the meat, spices and tomato paste. Thoroughly combine and cook until the minced beef is brown not pink.

7. Add some water, turn up the heat, then simmer on a lower heat for fifteen minutes, or until the water has disappeared.

8. You want your sauce to be quite dry. Set aside.

9. Turn up your oven to 400F / 200C.

10. Grease your baking dish with butter.

11. Combine the sour cream, mozzarella cheese and ⅔ of parmesan cheese. Season and add parsley.

12. In alternate layers build up your lasagne. Pasta sheet then meat sauce, pasta sheet then meat sauce.

13. Once they are all used up lay the cheese mix to the top spreading out evenly, sprinkle with the remaining parmesan cheese.

14. Cook in your oven for approximately thirty minutes. The cheese will be bubbling and golden brown.

15. Serve alongside a green salad and homemade dressing.

Autumnal Sausage and Pumpkin Soup

Serves 4 people

NUTRITION:
Ketogenic low carb
Per serving
Net carbs: 4 % (7 g)
Fiber: 2 g
Fat: 82 % (70 g)
Protein: 14 % (27 g)
kcal: 777

INGREDIENTS:

- 650 grams // 1 ½ lbs sausage meat
- 1 chopped red onion
- 1 diced small red pepper
- 1 minced garlic clove
- Pinch of salt
- ½ teaspoon dried sage
- ½ teaspoon dried thyme)
- 125 mls // ½ cup pumpkin puree
- 475 mls // 2 cups chicken broth
- 125 mls // ½ cup double cream
- 2 tablespoons salted butter

INSTRUCTIONS:

1. In a large frying pan cook the sausage meat, chopped onion and diced pepper.
2. Once the meat is cooked thoroughly, approximately fifteen minutes add the herbs, salt and pepper and mix.
3. Stir the broth in and add the cream and pumpkin puree.
4. On a low heat simmer for twenty minutes, the soup will thicken nicely.
5. Finish with adding your butter, serve immediately.

FOUR WEEK WEIGHT LOSS CHALLENGE

Use this handy four week plan to get you started. No cheating!

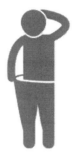

WEEK ONE

DAY ONE

BREAKFAST – PANCAKES, BERRIES AND CREAM (See page 24)

LUNCH – BROCCOLI AND KALE SALAD (See page 59)

DINNER –NO NOODLE CHICKEN AND CABBAGE SOUP

NUTRITION:
Ketogenic low carb
Per serving
Net carbs: 3 % (4 g)
Fiber: 1 g
Fat: 71 % (40 g)
Protein: 26 % (33 g)
kcal: 509

INGREDIENTS:

- 30 grams // 1 oz butter
- ½ tablespoon minced onion
- ½ chopped celery stalk
- 40 grams // ½ oz sliced mushrooms
- ½ garlic clove
- 475 mls // 2 cups chicken broth
- 15 grams // ½ oz diced carrots
- ½ teaspoon dried parsley
- ¼ teaspoon salt
- Pinch of black pepper
- 2 Cooked and shredded chicken thighs
- 35 grams // 1 ½ oz sliced green cabbage

INSTRUCTIONS:

1. In a large pan melt your butter on a medium heat.
2. Add your chopped celery, minced onion, garlic and sliced mushrooms. Cook for three to four minutes.
3. Pour in the chicken broth, carrots and parsley. Season and simmer until desired consistency of the vegetables you like.
4. Finally add your cooked chicken and the sliced cabbage.
5. Simmer for ten minutes more, the cabbage will be tender.

BREAKFAST – GINGER SMOOTHIE (See page 36)

LUNCH – BAKED BELL PEPPERS (See page 56)

DINNER – FRIED CHICKEN, BROCCOLI AND BUTTER

Serves 4 people

NUTRITION:
Ketogenic low carb
Per serving
Net carbs: 4 % (6 g)
Fiber: 3 g
Fat: 77 % (57 g)
Protein: 19 % (32 g)
kcal: 671

INGREDIENTS:

- 150 grams // 5 oz butter
- 650 grams // 1 ½ lbs boneless and skinless chicken thighs
- Salt & pepper
- 450 grams // 1 lb broccoli
- 1 small leek
- 1 teaspoon garlic powder

INSTRUCTIONS:

1. In your frying pan melt one half of your butter on a medium heat.
2. Season chicken and place into the frying pan. Cook for about twenty minutes in total, browning both sides. Remove and cover to keep warm.
3. Rinse the leek and broccoli and chop both into small size pieces.
4. Heat a separate frying pan and melt the rest of the butter, add your garlic powder and seasoning. Add leeks and broccoli and cook to al dente.
5. Serve together with your chicken and extra melted butter.

DAY THREE

BREAKFAST – ENGLISH MUFFINS (See page 38)

LUNCH – CAESAR SALAD

Serves 2 people

NUTRITION:
Ketogenic low carb
Per serving
Net carbs: 2 % (5 g)
Fiber: 3 g
Fat: 77 % (90 g)
Protein: 21 % (55 g)
kcal: 1060

INGREDIENTS:

Dressing

- 125 mls // ½ cup homemade mayonnaise
- 1 tablespoon Dijon mustard
- ½ lemon

- 20 grams // ¼ cup grated Parmesan cheese
- 2 tablespoons chopped anchovy fillets
- 1 chopped garlic clove
- Salt & pepper

Salad

- 350 grams // 12 oz chicken breasts
- Salt & pepper
- 1 tablespoon olive oil
- 75 grams // 3 oz bacon
- 200 grams // 7 oz chopped Romaine lettuce
- 40 grams // ½ cup grated Parmesan cheese

1. Turn your oven to 175C // 350F.

2. Whisk the dressing ingredients and set aside.

3. Put chicken breasts in your greased baking dish.

4. Season chicken and drizzle olive oil on top. Cook in the oven for twenty minutes or until fully cooked through.

5. Fry the bacon. Arrange lettuce as a base your plates. Top with sliced chicken and the crispy, crumbled bacon.

6. Finish with a generous dollop of dressing and a good grating of parmesan cheese.

DINNER – THAI FLAVOURED FISH CURRY (See page 64)

DAY FOUR

BREAKFAST – STRAWBERRY SMOOTHIE (See page 34)

LUNCH – SMOKED SALMON WITH AVOCADO (See page 46)

DINNER – CHICKEN SKEWERS WITH DIP AND FRIES

Serves 4 people

NUTRITION:
Moderate low carb
Per serving
Net carbs: 7 % (18 g)
Fiber: 5 g
Fat: 78 % (88 g)
Protein: 15 % (38 g)
kcal: 1030

INGREDIENTS:

Chicken skewers

- 800 grams // 1 ¾ lbs of boneless and skinless chicken thighs
- 1 teaspoon salt
- ¼ teaspoon black pepper
- 2 tablespoons olive oil
- 1 teaspoon garlic powder
- 1 teaspoon dried thyme
- 8 wooden skewers

Celery root fries

- 800 grams // 1 ¾ lbs swede or rutabaga
- 2 tablespoons olive oil
- ½ teaspoon salt
- ¼ teaspoon black pepper

Spinach dip

- 175 mls // ¾ cup homemade mayonnaise
- 4 tablespoons sour cream
- 2 tablespoons extra virgin olive oil
- 50 grams // 2 oz chopped frozen spinach
- ¼ teaspoon black pepper
- 2 tablespoons dried parsley
- 1 tablespoon dried dill
- 1 teaspoon onion powder
- ½ teaspoon salt
- 2 teaspoons lemon juice

INSTRUCTIONS:

1. Turn on the oven and set to 200C // 400F.

2. Place the salt, pepper, thyme, garlic powder and olive oil in a bowl and mix. Add chicken, coat thoroughly and let marinate for twenty minutes.

3. Peel the swede and cut into one cm pieces. Place them onto your baking tray lined with baking paper. Season and drizzle oil over and mix. Put into the oven for twenty minutes (you will cook them for longer though).

4. Push the chicken pieces onto skewers and place onto another baking tray lined in baking paper. Put them in the oven with your fries and cook both for half an hour. Check chicken is thoroughly cooked.

5. Make your dip by squeezing out extra liquid from spinach, then mixing in the rest of the dip ingredients.

6. Serve everything together.

DAY FIVE

BREAKFAST – EGG AND CHORIZO MUFFINS (See page 33)

LUNCH – GREEK SALAD

Serves 2 people

NUTRITION:
Moderate low carb
Per serving
Net carbs: 10 % (15 g)
Fiber: 5 g
Fat: 78 % (51 g)
Protein: 12 % (17 g)
kcal: 593

INGREDIENTS:

- 3 ripened tomatoes
- ½ cucumber
- ½ chopped red onion
- ½ green pepper
- 200 grams // 7 oz feta cheese

- 10 black olives
- 4 tablespoons olive oil
- ½ tablespoon red wine vinegar
- Salt & pepper

INSTRUCTIONS:

1. Cut up cucumber and tomatoes into small pieces.
2. Thinly slice the red onion and green pepper.
3. Arrange those vegetables on your plates.
4. Add olives and feta cheese, drizzle with the olive oil then the vinegar.
5. Season accordingly.

DINNER – PORK CHOPS AND BLUE CHEESE SAUCE (See page 68)

DAY SIX

BREAKFAST – OATMEAL (See page 35)

LUNCH – AVOCADO AND SEAFOOD SALAD (See page 49)

DINNER – LEEK AND BROCCOLI SOUP

Serves 4 people

NUTRITION:
Moderate low carb
Per serving
Net carbs: 8 % (10 g)
Fiber: 3 g
Fat: 81 % (50 g)
Protein: 11 % (15 g)
kcal: 545

INGREDIENTS:

Soup

- 1 leek
- 300 grams // ⅔ lb broccoli
- 475 mls // 2 cups water
- 1 vegetable stock/ bouillon cube
- 200 grams // 7 oz cream cheese

- 225 mls // 1 cup double cream
- ½ teaspoon black pepper
- 125 mls // ½ cup fresh basil
- 1 chopped garlic clove

Cheese chips

- 125 grams // 4 oz cheddar cheese
- ½ teaspoon paprika powder

INSTRUCTIONS:

1. Rinse and chop leeks finely. Cut the bottom core from the broccoli, slice thinly. Chop remaining broccoli florets into very small pieces.
2. Put these vegetables in a pan of water, add your stock cube, season and boil for two minutes, when the stem is soft.
3. Add the florets, turn down the heat and let simmer for three minutes. Check the broccoli is al dente.
4. Add the cream, black pepper, cream cheese, torn basil and garlic.
5. Using a handheld blender pulse the food until you get your desired consistency.
6. Add water if too thick, or cream if too thin.
7. Line a baking tray with parchment paper. Grate your cheese, place mounds onto the parchment. Leave 1 inch between.
8. Sprinkle each one with paprika.
9. Bake at 200C // 400F until the cheese has melted, about 5-6 minutes.
10. Eat alongside your soup.

BREAKFAST – KETO BREAD (See page 40)

LUNCH – OVEN BAKED BRIE

NUTRITION:
Ketogenic low carb
Per serving
Net carbs: 1 % (1 g)
Fiber: 1 g
Fat: 82 % (31 g)
Protein: 17 % (15 g)
kcal: 342

INGREDIENTS:

- 125 grams // 4 ½ oz Brie or Camembert cheese
- ½ chopped garlic clove
- ½ tablespoon fresh rosemary
- 30 grams // ¼ cup chopped pecans
- ½ tablespoon olive oil
- Salt & pepper

INSTRUCTIONS:

1. Turn on oven and set to 200C // 400F.
2. On a baking tray covered in baking paper place the cheese of your choice.
3. Mix together the chopped rosemary, garlic and pecans, add olive oil and season to taste.
4. Put this nut mix on top of the cheese.
5. Bake for ten minutes, cheese will be soft and nuts toasted.

DINNER – SWEDISH MEATBALLS (See page 70)

WEEK TWO

DAY EIGHT

BREAKFAST – BACON AND EGGS (See page 23)

LUNCH – STUFFED MUSHROOMS

Serves 2 people

NUTRITION:
Ketogenic low carb
Per serving
Net carbs. 4 % (6 g)
Fiber: 1 g
Fat: 86 % (51 g)
Protein: 10 % (13 g)
kcal: 526

INGREDIENTS:

- 110 grams // 4 oz bacon
- 6 mushrooms
- 1 tablespoon butter
- 125 grams // 4 oz cream cheese
- 1½ tablespoon chopped fresh chives
- ½ teaspoon paprika powder
- Salt & pepper

INSTRUCTIONS:

1. Turn oven on and set to 200C // 400F.
2. Grease with butter your baking dish.
3. Fry bacon until nice and crispy. Once cool crumble up and save the fat.
4. Remove your mushroom stems and chop them up finely, saute them in your bacon fat, add butter if necessary.
5. In a small bowl add your bacon bits and mushroom stems, cream cheese, chopped chives and paprika.
6. Lay out your mushrooms and fill each one with the mixture.
7. Cook for thirty minutes, the mushrooms will be a lovely golden-brown colour.

DINNER – GARLIC CHICKEN (See page 62)

BREAKFAST – STRAWBERRY SMOOTHIE (See page 34)

LUNCH – TORTILLA PIZZAS (See page 57)

DINNER – LAMB ROAST AND BROCCOLI PUREE

Serves 2 people

NUTRITION:
Moderate low carb
Per serving
Net carbs: 6 % (12 g)
Fiber: 4 g
Fat: 71 % (59 g)
Protein: 22 % (42 g)
kcal: 743

INGREDIENTS:

Lamb roast

- 325 grams // ¾ lb rolled lamb joint
- Salt & pepper
- 130 grams // ¼ oz cream cheese
- 2 tablespoons fresh thyme

- 1 garlic clove
- ¼ teaspoon lemon zest
- 25 grams // 1 oz butter
- cooking string

Broccoli purée

- 75 grams // ⅔ cup of Jerusalem artichokes
- 225 grams // 1 ½ lbs broccoli
- 35 grams // ⅓ cup butter
- ¼ teaspoon sea salt
- Pinch of black pepper

1. Turn on the oven and set to 160C // 320F.
2. Unroll the lamb onto your cutting surface. Season and spread your cream cheese onto it. Put herbs and garlic and zest from the lemon on it too.
3. Roll it all up and tie with your cooking string. Season the outside.
4. Put your meat into a greased baking dish.
5. Place an oven thermometer into thickest place in meat.
6. Cook until the core temperature has reached 60C // 140F. Or your desired cooking time.
7. Remove from oven and let rest.
8. While the meat is cooking you can make your puree.
9. Peel the artichokes and dice up into very small pieces. Boil for five to ten minutes in salted water.
10. Before the artichokes are cooked add the chopped up broccoli to the water and cook together.
11. Drain the pan, add butter and season.
12. Blend this mixture to a puree and serve with the lamb.

BREAKFAST – CREAMY COFFEE

NUTRITION:

Low carb

Per serving

Net carbs: 0 % (0 g)

Fiber: 0 g

Fat: 6 g

Protein: 0g

kcal: 100

INGREDIENTS:

◆ 1 cup coffee

◆ 60 mls // ¼ cup double cream

INSTRUCTIONS:

1. Make your coffee the way you like it. Pour the cream in a small pan and heat gently while stirring until it's frothy.

LUNCH – SMOKED SALMON WITH AVOCADO (See page 46)

DINNER – CHINESE STYLE PORK BELLY (See page 67)

DAY ELEVEN

BREAKFAST – COCONUT CREAM WITH BERRIES

NUTRITION:
Low carb
Per serving
Net carbs: (12.8 g)
Fiber: 3.9 g
Fat: 42 g
Protein: 4.6g
kcal: 446

INGREDIENTS:

- 125 mls // ½ cup coconut milk
- 50 grams // 2 oz fresh strawberries
- 1 teaspoon vanilla extract

INSTRUCTIONS:

1. Mix your ingredients in a blender and enjoy!

LUNCH – SUGAR SNAP PEA AND ROASTED FENNEL SALAD (See page 55)

DINNER – THAI FLAVOURED FISH CURRY (See page 64)

BREAKFAST – BANANA WAFFLES (See page 26)

LUNCH – TOFU SCRAMBLE

NUTRITION:
Moderate low carb
Per serving
Net carbs: 3 % (2 g)
Fiber: 5 g
Fat: 51 % (17 g)
Protein: 46 % (35 g)
kcal: 281

INGREDIENTS:

- 375 grams // 13 oz firm tofu
- ¼ teaspoon turmeric
- 1 tablespoon nutritional yeast
- 175 mls // ¾ cup unsweetened almond milk
- Salt & pepper
- 1 tablespoon chopped fresh chives

INSTRUCTIONS:

1. Break up your tofu in bite size pieces and add to a frying pan. Put the heat on medium, stir in turmeric and yeast and cook for five minutes.
2. Pour in almond milk and let simmer for ten minutes, stir occasionally. Season and garnish with your chopped chives.

DINNER – LASAGNE (See page 71)

DAY THIRTEEN

BREAKFAST – COCONUT PANCAKES (See page 25)

LUNCH – TURNIP GRATIN (See page 54)

DINNER – PARMESAN SALMON AND ASPARAGUS

Serves 2 people

NUTRITION:
Ketogenic low carb
Per serving
Net carbs: 4 % (6 g)
Fiber: 5 g
Fat: 69 % (51 g)
Protein: 27 % (45 g)
kcal: 680

INGREDIENTS:

- ◆ 450 grams // 1lb asparagus
- ◆ 1½ tbsp coconut oil, melted but not hot
- ◆ ½ teaspoon garlic powder
- ◆ 30 grams // 1 oz grated parmesan cheese
- ◆ 40 mls // ⅙ cup homemade mayonnaise
- ◆ ½ garlic clove
- ◆ 325 grams // ¾ lb boneless salmon fillets
- ◆ Dill for garnishing
- ◆ ½ slice of lemon

INSTRUCTIONS:

1. Turn on the oven to 175C // 350F.
2. Rinse the asparagus and trim the end of each spear.
3. Place the trimmed asparagus, coconut oil, and garlic powder in a plastic zip lock bag, seal, and shake lightly to coat asparagus.
4. In a small bowl, mix Parmesan cheese, homemade mayonnaise and garlic.
5. Lay out two rectangular pieces of baking paper, large enough to fit the asparagus and salmon, leaving plenty remaining on the sides and ends to fold into pockets and seal.
6. Divide the asparagus onto the sheets of baking paper.
7. Place the fillets on top, skin side down. Top the salmon with the homemade mayonnaise mixture.
8. Fold the baking paper over the fish and seal on all sides. Place the packets onto a baking tray and cook for twelve to fifteen minutes, the salmon will be slightly soft in the middle.
9. Garnish with fresh dill and lemon slices.

DAY FOURTEEN

BREAKFAST – ICED TEA
Serves 2

NUTRITION:
Ketogenic low carb
Per serving
Net carbs: 0 % (0 g)
Fiber: 0 g
Fat: 0 % (0 g)
Protein: 0 % (0 g)
kcal: 0

INGREDIENTS:

- 475 mls // 2 cups cold water
- 1 tea bag
- 225 mls // 1 cup ice cubes
- sliced lemon and fresh mint

INSTRUCTIONS:

1. Brew the tea and let it thoroughly cool. Remove the tea bag.
2. In a large jug add your ice cubes, tea, lemon and mint.
3. Top up with cold water and enjoy.

LUNCH – ANTIPASTO SALAD (See page 45)

DINNER – AUTUMNAL SAUSAGE AND PUMPKIN SOUP (See page 73)

WEEK THREE

DAY FIFTEEN

BREAKFAST – CHEESE ROLLUPS

Serves 2 people

NUTRITION:
Ketogenic low carb
Per serving
Net carbs: 2 % (2 g)
Fiber: 0 g
Fat: 82 % (30 g)
Protein: 16 % (13 g)
kcal: 331

INGREDIENTS:

- 110 grams // 4 oz sliced cheddar cheese
- 30 grams // 1 oz butter
- Paprika

INSTRUCTIONS:

1. Place your cheese slices onto your plate.
2. Spread butter onto the cheese, sprinkle with paprika and roll up. Nutrition.

LUNCH – GOATS CHEESE AND SPINACH PIE (See page 52)

DINNER – ORIENTAL STIR FRY WITH CABBAGE (See page 65)

DAY SIXTEEN

BREAKFAST – EGG AND CHORIZO MUFFINS (See page 33)

LUNCH – NO BREAD HERE SANDWICHES

Serves 1 person

NUTRITION:
Moderate low carb
Per serving
Net carbs: 5 % (5 g)
Fiber: 9 g
Fat: 84 % (34 g)
Protein: 11 % (10 g)
kcal: 383

INGREDIENTS:

- 50 grams // 2 oz of baby gem lettuce
- 15 grams // ½ oz homemade mayonnaise
- 30 grams // 1 oz edam cheese
- ½ sliced avocado,
- Four cherry tomatoes

INSTRUCTIONS:

1. Rinse your lettuce, spread the mayonnaise onto the leaves.
2. Layer the cheese, the avocado and tomato.

DINNER – COCONUT CURRIED CHICKEN (See page 63)

DAY SEVENTEEN

BREAKFAST – COCONUT PANCAKES (See page 25)

LUNCH – PESTO CHICKEN AND ZOODLE SALAD (See page 48)

DINNER – AUBERGINE // EGGPLANT GRATIN

Serves 2

NUTRITION:
Liberal low carb
Per serving
Net carbs: 12 % (14 g)
Fiber: 8 g
Fat: 74 % (38 g)
Protein: 14 % (16 g)
kcal: 485

INGREDIENTS:

- 450 grams // 1lb aubergine/eggplant
- 1 onion
- 1 tablespoon of butter or olive oil, for frying
- 75 grams // 2 ¾ oz feta cheese
- ½ tablespoon dried mint
- 10 grams // 1/6 cup chopped parsley
- 50 grams // 2 oz grated cheese
- 100 mls // 2/5 cup double cream
- Salt & pepper

INSTRUCTIONS:

1. Slice your aubergine/eggplant into one cm slices.
2. Brush on both sides with olive oil, sprinkle with salt and put onto your baking tray lined with baking paper.
3. Cook in the oven at 200C // 400F until nice and golden brown.
4. Meanwhile slice up your onion very thinly.
5. Put a frying pan on a medium heat and saute for about five minutes, season to taste.
6. Now to build your gratin. Put a layer of aubergine // eggplant in your baking dish, over the top place half of your cooked onions, the mint, parsley then two thirds of your feta cheese.
7. Add your final layer of aubergine/eggplant along with the remaining onion.
8. Sprinkle the rest of the feta cheese and then the grated cheese onto the top.
9. Lastly pour your cream over the whole dish and cook in the oven at 220C // 450F for thirty minutes. Your gratin will be golden and the cream bubbling.

DAY EIGHTEEN

BREAKFAST – CLOUD BREAD (See page 41)

LUNCH – ROAST BEEF WITH CHEDDAR CHEESE SALAD (See page 50)

DINNER – TAPAS PLATE

Serves 4

NUTRITION:
Ketogenic low carb
Per serving
Net carbs: 3 % (5 g)
Fiber: 1 g
Fat: 79 % (57 g)
Protein: 18 % (30 g)
kcal: 664

INGREDIENTS:

- 110 grams // 4 oz cheddar cheese
- 225 grams // 8 oz prosciutto
- 225 grams // 8 oz chorizo
- 125 mls // ½ cup homemade mayonnaise
- 110 grams // 4oz cucumber
- 50 grams // 2 oz red peppers

INSTRUCTIONS:

1. Cut the cold cuts and cheese into cubes. The vegetables into sticks.
2. Arrange on a plate. Enjoy!

DAY NINETEEN

BREAKFAST – CHAI TEA (See page 43)

LUNCH – FETA CHEESE WITH CHICKEN SALAD (See page 47)

DINNER – SEAFOOD CHOWDER

Serves 2

NUTRITION:
Ketogenic low carb
Per serving
Net carbs: 3 % (6 g)
Fiber: 1 g
Fat: 78 % (69 g)
Protein: 18 % (37 g)
kcal: 795

INGREDIENTS:

- 2 tablespoons butter
- 1 chopped garlic clove
- 75 grams // 2 ½ oz sliced celery
- 125 mls // ½ cup clam juice
- 175 mls // ¾ cup double cream
- 1 teaspoon dried sage
- ¼ lemon juice plus zest
- 50 grams // 2 oz cream cheese
- 225 grams // ½ lb white fish, bones removed
- 30 grams // 1 oz baby spinach
- 110 grams // 4 oz peeled, deveined shrimp
- Salt & pepper
- ¼ tablespoon red chili peppers

INSTRUCTIONS:

1. In a large pan on medium heat melt your butter.
2. Add your celery and garlic, cook for five minutes.
3. Pour the clam juice into the pot then add the cream cheese, cream, lemon juice and zest and sage. Simmer gently for ten minutes, stirring so it does not burn.
4. Add your choice of fish pieces and the shrimp. Simmer again for a few minutes until the fish is cooked.
5. Add the spinach and stir it until it wilts.
6. Season and garnish with the chilli if you want to.

DAY TWENTY

BREAKFAST – KETO BREAD (See page 40)

LUNCH – EGG MUFFINS

Serves 2

NUTRITION:
Ketogenic low carb
2 muffins per serving
Net carbs: 2 % (2 g)
Fiber: 0 g
Fat: 69 % (26 g)
Protein: 28 % (24 g)
kcal: 337

INGREDIENTS:

- 2/3 scallion, chopped
- 50 grams // 2 oz chopped chorizo
- 4 eggs
- 2/3 tablespoon red pesto
- Salt & pepper
- 50 grams // 2 oz grated cheese

INSTRUCTIONS:

1. Turn on the oven to 175C // 350F.
2. Grease a muffin tin.
3. Place scallions and meat inside each one.
4. Whisk your eggs together with the pesto and season. Mix in cheese.
5. Pour this into each muffin case.
6. Cook for fifteen minutes or until set.

DINNER – PORK CHOPS AND BLUE CHEESE (See page 68)

BREAKFAST – COCONUT PORRIDGE (See page 28)

LUNCH – COCONUT SALMON AND CABBAGE

Serves 2

NUTRITION:
Ketogenic low carb
Per serving
Net carbs: 2 % (4 g)
Fiber: 4 g
Fat: 81 % (68 g)
Protein: 17 % (33 g)
kcal: 768

INGREDIENTS:

- 275 grams // ⅔ lb salmon fillets
- ½ tablespoon olive oil
- 30 grams // 1 oz finely shredded coconut
- ½ teaspoon turmeric
- ½ teaspoon ground sea salt

- ¼ teaspoon onion powder
- 2 tablespoon olive oil
- 275 grams // ⅔ lb white cabbage
- 50 grams // 2 oz butter
- Salt & pepper

INSTRUCTIONS:

1. Cut up your salmon fillets into bite size pieces. Drizzle with your olive oil.
2. Mix up the shredded coconut with the onion powder, salt and turmeric on a plate, coat the salmon pieces in this.
3. In a frying pan on a medium heat saute your salmon until golden brown in colour.
4. Cut up your cabbage into wedges and saute in butter, they will be lightly caramelized. Season.
5. Serve your salmon with the caramelized cabbage and a wedge of lemon.

DINNER – CHICKEN SKEWERS WITH DIP AND FRIES (See page 79)

WEEK FOUR

DAY TWENTY-TWO

BREAKFAST – CAULIFLOWER HASH BROWN (See page 27)

LUNCH – CAULIFLOWER SALAD
Serves 2

NUTRITION:
Ketogenic low carb
Per serving
Net carbs: 4 % (5 g)
Fiber: 3 g
Fat: 91 % (51 g)
Protein: 5 % (6 g)
kcal: 512

INGREDIENTS:

Cauliflower salad

- 225 grams // 2 cups cauliflower
- Salt & pepper
- 40 mls // ⅙ cup water
- 50 grams // ⅓ cup bacon

- 1 celery stalk
- Small red onion
- ⅔ tablespoon fresh chopped chives

Dressing

- 125 mls // ½ cup homemade mayonnaise
- ¼ tablespoon Dijon mustard

- ¼ tablespoon cider vinegar
- Pinch of salt
- Pinch of black pepper

INSTRUCTIONS:

1. Preheat your grill to a low setting.
2. Cook in boiling water until soft.
3. Grill your bacon until nice and crispy.
4. In a large bowl add the cauliflower and crumbled bacon, the chives and diced onion.
5. Mix all your dressing ingredients and coat the cauliflower mix thoroughly.

DINNER – CHINESE STYLE PORK BELLY (See page 67)

DAY TWENTY-THREE

BREAKFAST – GRANOLA (See page 39)

LUNCH – ANTIPASTO SALAD (See page 45)

DINNER – CHICKEN PROVENCALE

Serves 2

NUTRITION:
Ketogenic low carb
Per serving
Net carbs: 2 % (5 g)
Fiber: 3 g
Fat: 82 % (94 g)
Protein: 15 % (39 g)
kcal: 1032

INGREDIENTS:

- 450 grams // 1lb grams chicken thighs
- 110 grams // 4 oz chopped tomatoes (fresh or tinned)
- 35 grams // 1 ¼ oz pitted black olives

- 2 tablespoons olive oil
- 2½ sliced garlic cloves
- ½ tablespoon dried oregano
- Salt & pepper

For serving

- 100 grams // 3 ½ oz lettuce
- 125 ml // ½ cup homemade mayonnaise
- ½ tsp paprika powder

- Zest of half a lemon
- Salt & pepper

INSTRUCTIONS:

1. Turn on your oven and set to 200C // 400F.
2. Put your chicken thighs into your baking dish and add the sliced garlic, black olives and tomatoes.
3. Drizzle generously with oil, sprinkle oregano and seasoning over the top.
4. Cook for approximately 50 mins, depending on chicken size pieces.
5. Serve with your salad and flavour your mayonnaise with lemon and paprika.

DAY TWENTY-FOUR

BREAKFAST – BANANA WAFFLES (See page 26)

LUNCH – AVOCADO AND SEAFOOD SALAD (See page 49)

DINNER – STEAK AND VEGETABLE KEBABS

Serves 2

NUTRITION:
Ketogenic low carb
Per serving
Net carbs: 4 % (14 g)
Fiber: 4 g
Fat: 81 % (128 g)
Protein: 15 % (55 g)
kcal: 1437

INGREDIENTS:

Marinade

- 125 mls // ½ cup olive oil
- 60 mls // ¼ cup soy sauce
- 1 tablespoon cider vinegar
- ½ teaspoon salt
- ½ teaspoon pepper
- 1 tablespoons of grated ginger
- 3 garlic cloves

Kebabs

- 450 grams // 1 lb sirloin steak
- 1 green pepper
- 1 red onion
- 225 grams // 8 oz mushrooms
- 4 skewers

1. Preheat the grill to medium.

2. In a small bowl, combine the ingredients for your marinade. Mix well. Set aside two tbsp of marinade into a smaller bowl.

3. Cut the steak into 1 to 2-inch cubes. Place them into the marinade coat well. Let sit for ten minutes.

4. Chop up the pepper, leave in big pieces. Cut onion in quarters. Cut mushrooms in half. Everything should be around the same size.

5. Build skewers by alternating meat, mushroom, bell pepper, and onion. Drizzle skewers generously with the already used marinade.

6. Place skewers under the grill, don't let them touch. Grill for 15-20 minutes, flipping every 5 minutes. When flipping, brush with reserved marinade.

DAY TWENTY-FIVE

BREAKFAST – STRAWBERRY SMOOTHIE (See page 34)

LUNCH – SMOKED SALMON WITH AVOCADO (See page 46)

DINNER – AUBERGINE // EGGPLANT PIZZA

Serves 2

NUTRITION:
Moderate low carb
Per serving
Net carbs: 8 % (13 g)
Fiber: 9 g
Fat: 69 % (50 g)
Protein: 23 % (37 g)
kcal: 671

INGREDIENTS:

- 1 aubergine/eggplant
- 40 mls // ⅙ cup olive oil
- 1 garlic clove
- ½ onion
- 175 grams // 6 oz minced beef
- 100 mls // ⅓ cup tomato sauce
- ½ teaspoon salt
- ¼ teaspoon pepper
- 150 grams // 1 ¼ cups grated cheese
- chopped fresh oregano

INSTRUCTIONS:

1. Turn on your oven to 200C // 400F.
2. Slice your aubergine/eggplant lengthwise to about 1cm in thickness.
3. Brush both sides with oil and put onto your baking tray already lined with baking paper. Cook for twenty minutes until just browning.
4. Chop up the garlic and fry it with the onion in oil until softened.
5. Add your minced beef and cook thoroughly, add your tomato sauce and seasoning. Simmer on low for ten mins, it will be nicely warmed through.
6. Once done take the aubergine/eggplant slices out of the oven and lay them flat onto the meat mix. Top with the cheese and oregano. Put back into the oven to melt the cheese.
7. Serve with green salad.

BREAKFAST – MICROWAVE OMELETTE

Serves one

NUTRITION:
Per serving
Net carbs: 0% (0 g)
Fiber: 0g
Fat: 69 % (50 g)
Protein: 23 % (37 g)
kcal: 190

INGREDIENTS:

- ◆ 1 egg
- ◆ 1 teaspoon cream cheese (full fat)
- ◆ 25 grams // 1 oz cheese

INSTRUCTIONS:

1. Crack the egg in a small bowl and add the cream cheese.

2. Mix well together.

3. Add the cheese and stir well.

4. Put in the microwave and heat on high power for 1 minute.

5. Enjoy!

LUNCH – AVOCADO AND SEAFOOD SALAD (See page 49)

DINNER – THAI FLAVOURED FISH CURRY (See page 64)

DAY TWENTY-SEVEN

BREAKFAST – SCRAMBLED EGGS MEXICAN STYLE (See page 31)

LUNCH – BROCCOLI AND KALE SALAD (See page 59)

DINNER – BACON WRAPPED MEATLOAF

Serves 4

NUTRITION:
Ketogenic low carb
Per serving
Net carbs: 2 % (6 g)
Fiber: 1 g
Fat: 79 % (90 g)
Protein: 18 % (47 g)
kcal: 1032

INGREDIENTS:

- 2 tablespoons butter
- 1 diced onion
- 650 grams // 1 ½ lbs minced pork
- 125 mls // ½ cup double cream
- 50 grams // 2 oz grated cheese
- 1 egg
- 1 tablespoon dried oregano
- 200 grams // 8 oz sliced bacon
- Salt and pepper

INSTRUCTIONS:

1. Turn on your oven to 200C // 400F.
2. Melt the butter over a medium heat in your frying pan, add the onions cook gently. Set aside.
3. Place the minced pork into a large bowl and add the cooked onions, and all the other ingredients except the bacon.
4. Form into the shape of your baking dish, wrap the loaf in the bacon.
5. Cook for about 50 mins, keep an eye on it as if the bacon looks overcooked the meat is done.
6. For a crispy bacon top place under the grill for a few mins.

BREAKFAST – OATMEAL (See page 35)

LUNCH – TUNA SALAD WITH EGGS

Serves 2

INGREDIENTS:

- 110 grams // 4 oz celery stalks
- 2 scallions
- 150 grams // 5 oz tuna in olive oil
- ½ lemon
- 125 mls // ½ cup homemade mayonnaise

- 1 teaspoon Dijon mustard
- 4 eggs
- 175 grams // 6 oz Romaine lettuce
- 110 grams // 4 oz cherry tomatoes
- 2 tablespoons olive oil
- Salt & pepper

INSTRUCTIONS:

1. Chop up the scallions and celery into fine pieces.
2. In a medium bowl mix the tuna, lemon juice, homemade mayonnaise, mustard, celery and scallions. Season and set aside.
3. Boil the eggs to your liking.
4. Divide the lettuce onto your plates, top with the tuna mix and eggs. Add the tomatoes and drizzle with olive oil.

DINNER – COCONUT CURRIED CHICKEN (See page 63)